Carb Cycling

The Ultimate Beginners Guide to Carb Cycling for Fat Loss

Table of Contents

Introduction

Congratulations! You have purchased a book that will guide you through everything you need to know about carb cycling and the impressive results this kind of diet can have on your body. Depending on what your specific personal goals are, this guide will help you make an informed decision as to whether a carb cycling diet is right for you and what kind of results you can expect with it.

In the coming chapters, we will be explaining the fundamentals and intricacies of carb cycling, and we'll take you through a basic training course on nutrition. You'll learn how different foods can affect your body weight and which carbohydrates are healthier than others.

We'll cover counting calories, explain how different foods react differently to your body and we will show you how to measure your caloric output versus intake and how carb cycling includes a scientific approach to dieting.

Once you're past the foundation of basic nutrition, you'll learn how to properly lay out a game plan before you engage in this kind of diet and how to navigate a cycled carbohydrate regimen successfully.

You'll also learn how to create, manage and customize your very own personalized diet and adjust it as your body changes, as well as different dietary approaches such as 'back loading,' in order to achieve specifically targeted results more quickly.

Losing excess body fat and improving muscle tone is the goal of millions of people around the world and everything a newcomer to carb cycling needs to know can be found on the following pages. You will learn how carbohydrates have gotten a bad reputation over the years, even though people cannot survive without them.

Carbs are the least understood part of the human diet, and we are going to help you understand the differences between simple and complex carbs, how they impact your body and what you can do about them.

You'll learn how all sugar is not created equally and we'll show you how changing your eating patterns can help you shed those excess pounds.

Carb cycling is one of the most popular diets around these days and for a good reason; it works! We understand that there are plenty of competing books on this subject, so thank you for purchasing this one. Enjoy!

Chapter 1
What Is a Carb Cycling Diet? Where Did It Come from and How Does It Work?

The birth of the carbohydrate reduced diet can be traced back to England in the 1860's. The first person known to attempt low carb dieting was a gentleman named William Banting.

Mr. Banting's story is one of a man tormented with the challenges of obesity who had discovered that no amount of exercise alone could rid him of his excess weight. For reference, he was just under five and a half feet tall and tipped the scales at a couple of hundred pounds.

Determined to tie his own shoes, he set upon a strict regimen of reduced carbs and successfully managed to lose a substantial quantity of body fat. Where an entire lifetime of physically demanding work and exercise had no impact on his weight, his committed attempt at a low carb diet resulted in the dramatic shrinking of his waistline.

The rest is diet history. Dieting strategies are constantly evolving, fads and trends fleet with time, but the ones that actually produce consistent, noticeable results quickly, are rare find indeed.

Carb cycling is one of these, essentially an evolution of the high protein, low carb diets that have become more popular over the past few decades, but with a twist. Yes, this diet does implement a lower carb approach to eating, but not in the traditional sense.

Historically, an Atkins inspired dietary approach leans toward increasing your protein and fat intake, in conjunction with lowering your carbohydrate consumption, while carb cycling takes things a step further by changing your percentage of carbohydrates on a daily basis.

This causes your body to focus on burning stored energy (body fat) while leaving your muscles and strength intact.

There are four primary components to carb cycling, and each has a minimal positive impact individually, however, when combined with the other three, can prove quite effective for reducing body fat without compromising muscle mass.

First, the bare essence of the carb cycling diet is getting your body to burn fat, rather than store it for reserve energy. Fat is literally your body's fuel storage system for emergencies, and by maintaining a consistent level of protein and fat consumption, combined with a scheduled manipulation of carbohydrate intake, you can alter and control the level of fat in your body.

Second, controlling the carbohydrate counts on your plate is only a small, yet important aspect of carb cycling. Altering your carb percentages during different days of the week also plays a major part of this dietary commitment. This is the 'cycle' part and requires some fundamental nutritional knowledge, which you'll read about in a coming chapter.

The third primary component is simply sticking to your guns and following through with your commitment. This can often be the most challenging part of the diet because a successful carb cycling campaign requires an above average level of commitment and strict adherence to the diet plan you'll be customizing for yourself. In other words, you have to walk the walk on this one.

The fourth and final component revolves around exercise and the timing of what, when and how much you eat. This is where you train your body to burn fat so that you can lose weight and improve muscle tone.

Carb cycling is a modernized and tweaked version of what William Banting first tried successfully in the mid nineteenth century. In the latter decades of the twentieth century, body builders and athletes began experimenting with this new cycling technique and quickly began to see exceptional results. Today, we live in an era where carb cycling combined with an exercise regimen is one of the most effective weight loss diets of all time and for a good reason; it works!

A diet that used to be exclusive to fitness professionals and competitors has now gone mainstream and due to its customized nature, can now be successfully utilized by anyone who is willing to follow this dietary and exercise routine.

The basic concept of carb cycling implements a seven-day routine where each day involves a pre-determined mix of exercise (or rest), in tandem with a managed carbohydrate intake. Some days are low carb, some are medium, and one or two are scheduled as high carb days.

By managing your diet this way, your body changes where it draws your energy from, pulling from your body fat while allowing your muscles to take everything they need.

The fact that cycling your carbohydrate consumption can be adapted to any schedule and lifestyle makes this type of diet very appealing. Instead of following a strict, yet boring low carb diet, carb cycling actually allows you to carb binge a little, once or twice a week. This is certainly a notable part of this diets successful reputation because it allows you to feed your cravings occasionally.

Carb cycling for fat loss is also unique in the sense that there is no single diet routine that everyone uses. Perhaps this is one of the better attributes as each person must develop and customize their own plan. In other words, by the time you are ready to actually begin cycling your carbs, you will have already become heavily vested in the diet because of the time and effort required to put a plan in place.

Another wonderful aspect of carb cycling is the fact that this is a temporary diet which produces measurable results quickly and rarely takes longer than eight or nine weeks. The appeal of fast results with only a temporary commitment can be a very compelling reason to give it a try.

The nature of carb cycling also allows you to test the waters with your toe before diving in, in the sense that early tweaking and adjustments are frequently required until you find the right mix of calories and carb intake for your body. No two carb cycling diets look the same, while the fundamentals remain equal for everyone.

Fans of carb cycling often refer to the ability to allocate one or two days per week for high carb meals as a huge selling point as this is one of the major drawbacks from an Atkins or Ketogenic style diet, which pushes you to avoid carbs at all cost. Let's be honest, carbohydrates not only taste great, but we also crave them on a regular basis. Just walking past a bakery and catching a whiff of freshly baked bread can drive a carb-starved individual mad.

Now that you have a rough idea of what carb cycling is, we move on to the important subject of nutrition basics and how different foods affect your body.

Chapter 2
Understanding Carbohydrates

It cannot be overstated how important it is to incorporate good eating habits into any diet and exercise routine. This is especially true for a carb cycling diet because you need to count your caloric input and output on a daily basis.

Engaging in just about any type of diet without having a reasonable grasp of basic nutrition is not a recipe for success. Since it cannot be assumed that all beginning dieters graduated Nutrition 101, we are going to give you a brief refresher course to help you along with your dieting plan.

This chapter exists mainly because a minimal amount of knowledge about nutrition, digestion and food groups is absolutely required if you are to have any chance of successfully carb cycling your body fat away. Our goal is to ensure you have every tool necessary to make the best decisions, however, please feel free to skip this chapter if you're already well versed in basic nutrition.

Everyone has heard of the food pyramid, and many people use it as a guideline for healthier eating. It has never been intended as a dieting tool but more of a guiding example of what a well-balanced diet might look like.

The one major shortcoming of the food pyramid is it does not address the individual differences that make us all unique. Some people have slower metabolisms; others burn more calories while exerting the same amount of physical energy. The point is not to undermine the food pyramid, but to make you aware that not all foods are equal, even if they fall into the same category.

By the end of this book, you should be able to make your own customized food pyramid. One that, if adhered to, can get you looking better and feeling healthier.

Nutritionally speaking, food falls into three primary categories: Fat, Protein, and Carbohydrates. Fat and protein are fairly straightforward and pretty much self-evident. Simply put, protein and fat are easily identifiable and not difficult to measure and count.

Carbohydrates, on the other hand, are more complicated since they are virtually everywhere and not so readily apparent. Fruits, vegetables, grains, legumes all contain carbohydrates in varying amounts. They also digest differently and break down into different types of sugars. Some have a propensity to become body fat, and these are the ones you want to avoid or reduce in your diet.

You need some of all three food types to survive, and carbohydrates are found in far more foods than you might think, but in the most basic sense, carbs are starches, fibers, and sugars. They are what makes things taste sweet, have good texture and nice visual appeal for example. Your body, however, digests granulated sugar differently than say, the sugar you might ingest from a bowl of ripe strawberries. It is what your body does with these different foods that make carbohydrates so unique and is why they deserve special attention when dieting.

Calories are simply the energy that is produced from food when digested. All food items contain a calorie by weight index, meaning a number of grams of x food item contain y number of calories. It is these caloric indexes that allow you to measure a diet.

What this boils down to is when you consume calories, they are going to break down in your digestive system and convert into energy. If you burn as many calories as you ingest, your weight is going to be maintained, more or less. If you consume fewer calories than you burn, you will lose weight, and the opposite will happen if you ingest more calories than you use.

Protein and fat give you calories, but your body does not generally use these for stored energy (body fat) unless you consume more than your body requires. Carbohydrates, on the other hand, tend to gravitate towards the fat in your body, storing that energy for a rainy day. This is particularly true with fructose and sucrose, the simple sugars.

Sugar, fiber, and starch are the three words used to best describe carbohydrates. However, not all carbs are created equal. Some are simple, and some are more complex.

Simple carbs are usually found in food items which contain higher levels of sweetness, from ripened fruit to pastries, for example. These are the sugars that easily become body fat if you consume more than you burn. They are also the sugars that give you a fast energy burst because they digest quickly into the bloodstream and tend to burn off quickly or stow away as excess body fat. You will also recognize these types of carbs like the ones that seem to fill your stomach quickly but find yourself hungry a short time later. Chinese fast food is infamous for this and probably the best-known example.

Complex carbs, on the other hand, are found in grains, vegetables, beans and so on. Generally, the higher the fiber and starch content, the more complex the carb. Mainly due to the fiber presence, these sugars and starches digest more slowly, and your body burns more calories during the digestive process, so you will know them as foods that typically keep you full for a longer period of time. Rich, creamy pasta is a well-known example of this.

Basically, carbs that fall into the complex category are healthier than the simple ones, but this is not exclusive since your body needs a variety of nutrients from different food sources. Balancing your diet is just as important as paying attention to what you eat.

Identifying the simple carbs from the complex carbs is the first thing you need to know when attempting to manage your diet, so here is a brief list for reference. You should notice that the simple carbs are most commonly found as ingredients in processed foods while the complex carbs are present in more natural, wholesome foods.

Simple carbs:

- Sugary products

- Sodas

- Ripe fruit and juices

- Pastries

- White bread

- Cereals

- Chips

Complex carbs:

- Vegetables

- Grains

- Nuts

- Legumes

- Wheat bread

- Oats

Ingredient and nutrition labels are fairly reliable tools for helping you identify which foods to avoid or minimize and there is one time tested measure that makes this even easier; 'The more ingredients on the label, the higher the amount of simple carbohydrates.'

There is no way to completely avoid eating all carbohydrates, and you would not remain healthy if you tried. On any given day, your diet is going to contain around sixty percent of carbs with the rest being protein and fat. It is which ones you choose to consume that matters and how much of them you eat. In other words, carbohydrates are not as bad as you've heard, in fact, you need them.

It is also important to know when the best time is to eat certain carbs and the best times to avoid them. This is a huge part of successful carb cycling, and we'll get into greater detail on this later in the book.

Now that you have a better grasp of what carbohydrates actually are let's take a look at how calories come into play.

Chapter 3
Understanding Calories

Any and every diet you consider is going to involve counting the calories you ingest and measuring the calories you burn off. There are plenty of smartphone apps available that can calculate this for you easily. However, a little understanding of caloric fundamentals can go a long way towards helping your dietary endeavors become a success story.

One important component of creating your own carb cycling regimen is getting a solid grasp on exactly how many calories your body uses up on any given day. Obviously, if you are an individual who works out at the gym three times a week, but sits behind a desk at work all day, you burn more calories on workout days than you do on rest days.

Before you can focus on carb cycling or any diet, you need to identify your own burn rate. This will take a little effort, but once you know this, setting your goals of body fat loss becomes much easier.

A calorie is a unit of measure much like a measuring spoon or cup, except it measures potential energy of food if consumed and used up during physical activity. For example, walking one mile can burn 100 calories of energy, while eating a pear can give you 100 calories of energy. So a pear becomes a mile you need to walk to have a net gain of zero. This is just one way a savvy dieter can analyze a plate at dinner.

As previously mentioned, calories are measurements of potential energy consumed. They are found in every single food we consume, to varying degrees. This discovery goes back over two hundred years, credited to the 17th-century chemist, Wilbur Atwater.

It is Atwater who discovered what is known as the 4-9-4 method of measuring potential energy in different foods. What he found was that fat, as in the marbling you might find on a steak, contains over twice the amount of calories you would find in an equal amount of lean protein or carbohydrates.

Using the metric system, Atwater's results show that one gram of protein has approximately four calories, as does one gram of carbs, while fat contains somewhere in the neighborhood of nine calories in just one single gram.

While these 4-9-4 numbers are derived from science, there are a million variables involved, so consider these a rough estimate of calories, not an exact, indisputable fact. Potential energy and actual energy retrieved, will rarely match up with simple things like how well something is chewed can have a huge impact on how much energy your body is able to absorb from any given food item.

This variable estimation actually helps you in a carb cycling regimen because your body learns to pull as many calories as possible from your diet, allowing your body to require less food to get by as time passes.

A caloric baseline is a number of calories your body needs to maintain your weight. If you are gaining weight on a regular basis, your caloric intake is too high. But what is the magic number of calories to just maintain a level body weight? This number is your baseline and can only be determined by you. Even a person who has the exact same weight and height as yourself will have a different baseline than you.

Yes, there are averages and recommended calorie levels available for reference, and usually, these are based on sex, weight, and height. The problem is that they do not take into account important factors such as lifestyle, metabolism, and more importantly, what you actually eat. The variables here are endless.

A huge part of a successful carb cycling diet is knowing your own body and what you need. You cannot control whether an apple has exactly 92 or 106 calories, so you must depend on averages. However, with your own body, you can really dial into specifics. It just takes a little work and practice.

The reason we are bringing this up now is that carb cycling for fat loss is a diet approach that requires a large degree of commitment and attention to detail. It is not the type of diet one jumps into, like a cold pool. In fact, it is just the opposite, and every serious carb cycler will tell you the same exact thing; work your way slowly into this diet, it is not for everyone and takes a lot of focus on details, but the results can be amazing.

So, knowing your caloric baseline is a good first step because this is going to help you decide how many carbs you'll need to reduce, once you commit to the diet. Get in the habit early of reading labels, counting calories and writing down your intake and weight on a daily basis.

The best way to figure out your magic calorie number is to start a fitness diary and begin counting the calories you consume on a daily and recording your weight right alongside. This is also a great way to ease yourself into tracking where you are and where you'll begin training yourself to burn off your body fat.

Start counting calories and adjust your intake weekly until you find that your weight has 's flattened out to a stable number. No need to adjust the variety in your diet yet, just the amount of calories. Play around with this, it can be a lot of fun! Consider it a pre diet dress rehearsal where the results aren't nearly as important as the practice itself.

Once you get to a stable weight and know how many calories your body needs to stay there, then you will be ready to start cycling your carbs and begin shedding body fat.

Your fitness diary will come in very handy down the road once you begin filling it with daily details and results. Especially when you have enough information to begin aggregating and identifying patterns. There are many dieting apps available to assist you with this as well. You will find this to be extremely valuable information after just a few weeks of carb cycling.

In summary, before you delve into carb cycling, train yourself to get in the habit of reading, counting and writing down calorie intakes and weight changes on a daily basis. It is also recommended that you try one or two different types of carbo-centric diets before attempting to cycle your carb intake. In other words, this is not your very first diet kind of diet.

Chapter 4
Understanding Protein and Fat

Protein is probably the most common thing that people understand about food. Ask anyone to name a protein, and you'll immediately hear the words meat, steak, fish, etc.

Ask the same question while substituting the word fat for protein and you enter into a whole new realm of facials expressions. The awful truth is that fat is misunderstood because the word has different meanings, depending on context. Body fat, dietary fat, fatty acids, trans fat, unsaturated fat, saturated fat. It can be confusing.

Consuming fat does not necessarily increase a person's body fat. Fat does not migrate towards other fat. These are common myths and fat has a deserved place at the table, so let's explore further.

Body fat is stored energy. Fat in food from plants or animals is also stored energy, but they are not the same. More often than not, consuming fat is not even a static weight contributor, unless you are consuming larger quantities than you need.

Everyone has heard of professional athletes who boast of extremely low body fat levels. Many of these individuals strive for extremely low-fat counts, generally for an upcoming competitive event, such as boxing, for example, where every ounce counts. In these cases, what has happened is the athlete had focused on converting every possible ounce of body fat into muscle for an upcoming competitive event. This is always a temporary goal for a specific event, and most athletes revert back to normal body fat levels after a competition is completed.

This alone should tell you that body fat doesn't have to be a bad thing and also maintaining extremely low levels of body fat can actually be harmful to your health. The fact is we need fat as it is considered a macro nutrient, meaning it should make up a decent part of your diet, to promote good health.

Body parts that depend on fat include the brain, the eyes, the liver and many other organs. Think about this; the organs that we use to think, to see and to filter our blood need fat. Nobody is recommending that you remove fat from your diet. However, all nutritional experts agree that managing your total fat intake is a critical part of a healthy lifestyle. What is just as critical, however, is paying attention to what types of fat you consume and which ones you should try to avoid.

Managing your level of body fat can definitely be a good thing, and carb cycling can certainly help with this. In fact, there aren't many diets out there that perform better than carb cycling to reduce body fat. Understanding different types of fat, knowing which ones you need and avoiding the ones you don't can really have a significant impact on your dieting success, so let's take a closer look at them.

Most doctors and nutritionists recommended that the fat in your diet should fall around ten percent of your daily calories, but not more. More importantly, these fat calories should come from natural sources, rather than processed foods. Basically, you will find good fats in foods where it is naturally present, and you will find bad fats in foods where it has been added.

Generally, fats are categorized into different types, such as saturated fat, unsaturated fat and trans fat.

Unsaturated fats are the best kinds to ingest as they tend to be the ones that make your body system function smoothly, are easily digested and quickly put to good use. You will find these good fats in most cold water seafood and avocados. Omega 3 fatty acids, for example, are found in abundance in salmon.

The opposite is true of saturated fats and trans fatty acids. These are the fats that go to the places you don't want them and tend to stay there. Other than providing calories for conversion to energy, they don't do a whole lot of good for you, nutritionally speaking.

Saturated and trans fats are easily recognizable as they are not found in liquid form at room temperature. Hydrogen is usually added to these oils to keep them in solid form at room temperate, ostensibly for visual appeal and shelf life.

Ever wonder why a packaged pastry at the convenience store looks so good, even though it has likely been around for quite a while? It's the bad kind of fat, that's why. It looks great and doesn't go bad, sometimes ever! The uneducated consumer is more interested in how good something looks and how yummy it tastes, rather than being focused on whether it is healthy or not.

Manufacturers understand this consumer attitude well, and the retailer simply does not want to have to deal with throwing away expired pastries every day. This is the world we live in today and any dieter who pays attention to what they eat, is essentially them an enemy of the processed food empire.

We're going to try and make this easy for you. As a general rule, if you prepare your own meals, there won't be a lot of saturated and trans fats involved. If your diet is based around prepared, or heat and serve type meals, you are going to be ingesting more bad fats than your body needs and these fats will store themselves away as body fat.

We talked earlier in this book about how a carb cycling diet typically includes adjustments on your daily carbohydrate intake while maintaining a relatively flat line of calories from protein and fat. Even though you might be rationing your daily fat intake to ten percent of your diet, for example, the key here is to maximize your good fat intake while minimizing your bad fat exposure.

Keeping it simple is the main secret ingredient on the menu to body fat loss. Preparing your own meals will naturally help you avoid the bad fats while consuming processed and manufactured foods will increase your body fat level of the fats you are trying to avoid.

Chapter 5
Planning for Carb Cycling

There is a reason why you're here and reading this book right now. Maybe you planned it, or perhaps you just made the decision on a whim. Regardless, here we are. That might work for reading a book or stopping by a fast food joint for a snack, but it definitely won't work for a carb cycling diet. Not a chance.

Of all the different options for dieting available, carb cycling is certainly one of the most planning and detail intensive kind you will encounter. Why is that?

Well, the most obvious reason is that cycling your carb intake alone is not as effective as merging your carb cycles with a regular workout routine. While it is possible to reduce your body fat by carb cycling alone, the best results come with the timing of when you ingest your carbs, how many you consume and how quickly you burn them off.

If you recall, we previously discussed how sugar, fiber, and starch are all forms of carbohydrates and that sugars are absorbed more quickly while fiber and starch take some time to digest.

Whenever you consume sugar while remaining inactive for a period of time, since you're not burning off that sugar, your body is going to store it in the form of body fat for a rainy day. Remember, the sugary parts of carbohydrates get absorbed quickly, which means they are also the fastest calories to become fatty tissue. It also takes very little energy for this to happen, so you're burning fewer calories just to digest what you've eaten. Therefore, the net punishment on your body is noticeably higher than starchy carbs. The digestive system has to work for its food, burning calories to get energy from calories in starchy and high fiber foods.

One important key to successful carb cycling is taking in your essential carbohydrates when your body is most likely to use them immediately for nutritional purposes rather than for energy storage. This is one of the main reasons why planning is such an important aspect here.

Many carb cycling diet plans have three days a week of low carb intake, three days of mid-level carbs and one day of 'carbo-heaven.' Body builders and fitness professionals seem to swear by the on, off, on, off, on, off, then carbo-heaven rotation and spend their gym time on the higher carb days while resting on, the lower carb days. Not only does this help reduce body weight fat by burning more calories on higher calorie days, but it also reduces the available calories for fat on rest days.

If you think about it, this would be very difficult to achieve without having planned ahead. Having a readily accessible calendar and spending a few minutes planning it out each week will go a long way in contributing to your conquering of body fat.

It's not just the gym schedule you need to map out, but also your meals. In a future chapter, we discuss the importance of learning to prepare your own meals as not only can this save you a ton of money and be very rewarding, but it also allows you to dial in on what is really going into your body as opposed to what you 'think' is going into your body.

Once you've determined what your caloric baseline is and what your diet targets are, it's time to crunch some numbers and put them on the calendar.

From a calorie standpoint, assuming three meals per day, you'll want to schedule your total of 21 meals per week all at the same time. There are multiple reasons for this, but the most obvious is simplicity. It's a lot easier to map out seven-morning meals at once rather than waking up and wondering what's for breakfast.

This is also when you should be doing some reverse math and catering your menu towards the desired calories in any given day part.

To keep things easy and consistent, many carb cycling dieters will map out the exact same breakfast and lunch for an entire week, while using dinner time to alternate between higher and lower carb meals. This is easier for shopping, easier for portion control, easier for meal preparation and produces less food waste. It also makes it easier for you to follow through with your plan.

So be prepared to plan your meals ahead, one full week in advance and set your higher carb days around your exercise schedule. It is also a good practice that helps you develop the habit of following through with commitments and actually going to the gym when you originally planned to.

Chapter 6
Easing Your Way into Carb Cycling

Trying to shock your body into losing weight is a story that rarely finishes with a happy ending. When people first hear about the concept of carb cycling for fat loss and read stories about some who experience tremendous results quickly, it is natural to want all that fat gone now. The key point here is to keep your goals realistic and achievable.

Taking baby steps not only allows your body to prepare and adjust to the changes you will experience, but it also allows you to prepare for the changes in your eating pattern mentally. One of the most common mistakes made in any diet is setting the bar too high and then getting discouraged when the set goals are not reached. It cannot be stressed enough; go low, slow and steady, building your way towards a full on carb cycling schedule.

The truth is that anyone who jumps hardcore on the carb cycling bandwagon without gearing up for it first and letting your body adjust is putting their health at risk. Those who do go from zero to a hundred in lickety-split are usually people who have some sort of competition around the corner and are willing to put their long term health aside for the benefit of near term gain. Most people, and especially beginners, will want to avoid this approach as the risks will likely outweigh the rewards.

If you do indeed decide it is a risk you are willing to take because of an upcoming event that is that important to you, be certain to talk with your doctor first, even though they will certainly advise you against it. In fact, it is always advisable to consult with your doctor regarding any significant dietary changes, before you engage in them. Your doctor is certainly the most qualified person to offer advice and guidance on this subject.

Dropping your carbohydrates quickly or too much can kill you. Literally. This is why it is so critically important that you work your way through a transition period. As a rule of thumb, this works on both ends of the spectrum, on your way into the diet and on your way out

A typical window for a full on carb cycling diet is somewhere around eight or nine weeks long. Some people achieve their desired results in a shorter period of time. However, the general consensus is never longer than nine weeks. You are taxing your system in ways that your body is not used to, which can lead to both short and long term health issues.

Now seems like a good time to explain that carb cycling for fat loss is a temporary diet and is never recommended as a full-time lifestyle. Reducing your excess carb intake for health reasons is one thing, depriving yourself of them is a whole different matter entirely and can result in a myriad of health related issues. This is a diet that you need to take seriously and pay attention to details. The implications for not doing so can be severe.

It is advisable to allow two weeks of transitioning yourself into carb cycles, not just so that your digestive system can adjust but also allow yourself to demonstrate you are willing to tend to all the details involved. Remember, this is a detail intensive diet, so the more prepared you are, the greater your chance of success.

If you're not counting calories, if you're not using a scale to weigh your food, if you're not writing out a weekly menu and gym schedule and actually following through, then this diet is simply not for you. It won't work. The transition time will allow you to figure this out and make good decisions. This is ultra-critical if it's your first attempt at carb cycling.

Body builders and certain athletic competitors only use carb cycling leading up to a competition, then revert back to more conventional diet routines afterwards. The eight or nine-week timeline referenced above is just enough time to alter your digestive system, lose excess body fat and convert remaining body fat to muscle.

Once this is achieved, continuing to cycle your carbohydrates has little benefit but does pose increased risk to health and may create some deficiencies of nutrients. These can cause serious, long term problems, to virtually every part of your body.

So plan to slide in gradually over a couple of weeks, get your routine set, hit your goals and get out. This is that kind of diet. For many people, carb cycling is ideal once a year, in the springtime, gearing up for the summer beach season. For others, they just want to get down to a specific weight or body shape, so that they can focus on simply maintaining their weight. The good news is that cycling your carbs can work for both end goals and often does.

One final thought on the importance of taking your time, as you work into a carb cycling routine; you will likely experience some degree of subtle body changes, such as lower testosterone levels while experiencing an increase in stress. By changing your diet incrementally, your body has time to adapt, and the impact will be far less noticeable. If nothing else, your friends, family, and coworkers will appreciate this.

Chapter 7
Good Carbs, Bad Carbs, and Ugly Carbs

Carbohydrates sure have gotten a bad rap lately. It seems like everyone hates them more than ever. This is unfortunate because they are often misunderstood. Many of the nutrients your body needs only originate from carb heavy foods, and as a general rule, over half your caloric intake should be in the form of carbohydrates, and up to 70% of those should be complex carbs. We won't survive without them, so trying to avoid them outright is not a good idea.

Let's take a look at the good carbs. They are complex, they have fiber, they have starch, and they taste good. So where on your plate can you typically find the good guys in the carb gang? In your salad, but maybe not your salad dressing.

Leafy greens? Check. In fact, just about anything green is going to be one of the good guys. Asparagus, broccoli, bell peppers, green onions, okra, jalapeños, spinach.

Oil and vinegar type dressings are generally very low in carbs, while creamy dressings can contain quite a bit. They're both okay, just go light on the creamy stuff during your low carb meals.

The good news is that even on low carb days, you can put away a good amount of green salad with your protein without maxing out on your daily carb ration. You get a really good bang for your buck when filling up on the complex carbs.

You get a good amount of fiber, very little sugar, and a reasonable quantity of starch. Since carb cycling generally avoids zero carb days like some diets, you can flavor your salads up with beets, berries or other naturally sweet foods and still maintain a good balance of complex and simple carbohydrates.

What else is good? Beans, root veggies, brown rice, grains. steamed cauliflower, broccoli, carrots, fresh herbs.

These are all on the top shelf in the carb store. Basically, any vegetable that is low in sugar but high in starch and fiber is going to be on the good list. One super good item you wouldn't expect to find on this list is bananas that have not ripened yet. The starches haven't turned to sugars yet, and the fiber is off the charts. This also applies to several other fruits before they ripen. Think of it this way; the naturally sweeter an item, the more quickly those sugars enter your blood stream while the less sweet, the slower they enter your blood stream. Slower equals better when it comes to carbohydrates and digestion, with regards to body fat.

These items make the good list because you can eat about as much as you want while carb cycling. The point here is that your stomach would fill up before you have maxed out on your daily carb ration.

Okay, so what's the bad stuff and where might you find it on your plate?

Bad is probably not the best word to use here because it's ambiguous. It is really more about how much is too much, as a limited amount of bad is not really bad at all. In fact, it can be good, just not good enough to eat as much as you want. You'll want to manage how much of these carbs you ingest while cycling, but no need to avoid them entirely.

Usually, you will encounter these items presented as side options. A baked potato, rice, ripened fruit, corn, salsa, fruit bowls and things of that nature. Basically, side dishes that are minimally processed. Pasta, risotto, and even broth based soups are pretty decent but certainly not in stews, gravies and thickened sauces. With all this said, keep in mind that when it comes to food and health, variety is key to good health, diet or no diet, as long as you avoid or minimize the ugly stuff.

So what is the ugly stuff and where will you likely find it on your plate?

It is not always easy to completely avoid the ugly carbs. However, these are definitely the ones you want to pay the closest attention to.

Just about anything mass produced in a food facility that ends up in a package where all you need to add is water or milk is going to be on this list. Look at the ingredient label, and if it contains more than four or five ingredients, this is where you start encountering modified corn syrup and such. The closer an ingredient is to the top of an ingredient label, that means it is a higher percentage of the overall content. By law, ingredient labels must be presented in descending order of content, by weight. As a simple example, all natural lemonade should contain only three ingredients. Water is the majority ingredient, followed by sugar, then lemon juice.

Any time you see corn syrup in the top six items of an ingredient label, keep on walking. The main reason this item is found in so many products is cost. It is less expensive than sugar and far less healthy.

Anything heavily processed or shelf stable when you know it shouldn't be, deserves close scrutiny. Wonder bread, cookies, donuts, pastries, candy bars, soda, energy drinks, flavored drinks that don't qualify as juices, etc. Now you should understand why the filling inside an oreo cookie never melts when left in your car on a hot day. It reacts similarly inside your body in the sense that it just doesn't want to go away.

Why are cereals fortified with vitamins C and D these days? It is not for the children's sake, unfortunately. It is there in the hope that mom will see it on the front of the box and not bother reading the 37 ingredients on the label. This is a subject that is not written about enough when dieting and health are the discussions. The distractions on the cover of food packaging are designed to catch your eye but are also created with the hope that you won't read the ingredients. Don't be fooled!

If it resembles anything like a dessert from grandma's kitchen or could be a distant cousin of junk food, then make every attempt to forgo these for a couple of months while you're cycling. In terms of body fat, this is, by far, your worst enemy. These are the items heavy in simple carbohydrates and sweetening additives that want to migrate directly to your body fat and hang out for a couple of decades. However, just because something is sweet does not make it bad for you. Focus on where the sweetness is coming from.

Remember, simple carbs are sugars, equal easy fat, and fast energy while complex carbs make your body work harder for the nutrients and energy contained inside of you. The more complex carbs require a significantly larger amount of energy to break down and digest, so essentially they are giving you a head start in the calorie burning department.

Chapter 8
Determining If Carb Cycling is Right for You

Every diet has side effects and the more information you have available, the better decisions you can make as to whether a specific one is right for you.

The most famous side effect of carb cycling is fat loss, and it's no coincidence that this is also the main reason why people engage in it. It is not, however, the only effect of carb cycling, nor is it the only reason why people try this diet.

As we pointed out earlier in this book, the invention of carb cycling resulted from the professional body building industry back in the 1980's. Essentially, after ten months of regular workouts focusing on all the different muscles of the body, building up strength and muscle tone, carb cycling for the last eight or nine weeks really honed in on losing any excess body fat and enhancing the tone of competitive body builder's muscles. That little extra edge which might give them any slight advantage over others. Every trick in the book would be tried and no physical expense spared. Sometimes those side effects were worth it, since winning the competition was a more important short term goal than any longer lasting issues which arose.

Some of these effects are physical and some lean more towards the emotional side of things. This is why it is so critically important for anyone considering a carb cycling diet to not only understand as much about the process as possible but also for see some of the side effects and ensure they don't carry over into your daily life outside of diet and exercise.

One significant side effect of carb cycling can be a strong feeling of hunger on your lower carb days. That is the physical side effect, but it comes with an emotional side effect, as well, and that is being miserable or difficult to be around. Your stress levels increase, and you can find yourself being completely consumed by cravings for starchy or sugary foods. It can literally become the only thing on your mind and distract you away from other important things in your life. There is nothing glorious in losing friends on a diet.

Remember, carbs are generally the foods that give you the full stomach feeling, so it's logical that you would experience some hunger on low carb days. However, if your work profession is customer service, for example, how do you think you would perform your duties if you were miserably hungry? You might look great at work, but you might not have a job for long. Or your coworker's might not like being around you and complain to your boss. These are potential consequences that should not be ignored.

There are endless scenarios here, and the thing is people sense when others around them are unhappy, or grumpy, or whatever. As human beings, we are not good at concealing this, and we are quite effective at picking up these types of signals from others. If you are in a position where your mood can have a dramatic impact on your employability status, you'll need to take this into consideration when thinking about carb cycling. Experiencing an increase in stress is not uncommon either. Usually, it is temporary. However, it is stress and is something will possibly be noticed in your work. Be aware of this potential hazard and adjust accordingly.

That does not mean you should avoid this diet at all costs, just that you should consider your carb cycle scheduling and maybe ensure your low carb days only fall only on your days off. There are other creative ways you can still carb cycle effectively, without it affecting your work life. An example of this might be taking in carbohydrates for breakfast and lunch all your days, going to no carb dinners, thus avoiding this potential side effect during business hours.

Mood swings and grumpiness are just one of the potential side effects. Another is energy level swings, especially during the early stages of your diet, as the body and the digestive system begin to change and adjust. You may also experience swings in your insulin levels as well.

The human body has this strange attribute where after years of poor eating habits, it feels like it wants to fight you against changing to good eating habits. This is most true during the transition to burning stored body fat. It takes several days, if not a few weeks to get used to this and can be one of the most challenging parts to endure during the early phase of carb cycling. It can be manageable and is more easily dealt with if you know what to expect, so keep this in mind.

As another example, if your work requires a high level of physical exertion and concentration for long periods of time, it is almost certainly best to avoid putting yourself in a bad situation on the job, so try to work around it, if at all possible, with your diet schedule.

For pregnant women or women who may be about to get pregnant, a carb cycling diet is an absolute no. It can be extremely unhealthy for both you and your baby, even fatal sometimes. There are so many dramatic changes happening during pregnancy, adding the confusion of a changing diet can lead to a number of problems, including misdiagnosis of the cause of potential medical concerns. Save your carb cycling considerations for getting back to your pre mom body afterwards. It is just not worth the risk. Besides, you'll have enough going on in your life for the time being.

People with type II diabetes should also avoid carb cycling as this can tax your body and result in even more unpredictable blood sugar levels, making your diabetes difficult to manage and treat. It can also send you into diabetic shock by making your body alter its insulin production due to the fact that carb cycling is effective as a dietary system by changing a number of available sugars in your blood.

So who should try carb cycling? The simple answer is anyone who is generally in good health and desires to lose some excess body fat. It can be a fantastic diet for runners, swimmers, people who regularly go to the gym or frequently work out at home and, of course, body builders.

Cycling your carbs can also be a great diet for people who work in demanding jobs where you burn a lot of calories but just can't seem to arrive at your ideal body weight. In this case, burning your calories is not the problem, eating too much is. This is the kind of diet that teaches you how to eat better by forcing you to pay attention to what kinds of foods you eat.

Carb cycling does not require you exercise in order for it to be an efficient body fat trimmer, it just helps increase the shrinkage of your fat. For someone who wants to drop an inch or two around the waist without having to commit to a gym membership, this diet does work, although you'll miss out on the natural improvement of muscle toning that naturally occurs if you do both together.

Chapter 9
Mapping Out Your Game Plan

Now that you have a reasonably good idea what carb cycling is and how it can help you to lose body fat, it is time to start looking at a cycling plan that you can work with.

You are going to need some tools to help map out your plan. A digital scale that measures in grams, a calendar that you can write on and a daily calendar that you can use as a diary of sorts, to track your progress. Fortunately, in this age of the smart phone, dozens of apps are available to help with this as well and make tracking as easy as texting.

Every body is unique in its own way, so it is crucial to focus on yourself and set your goals realistically. Fundamentally, dieting revolves around calories, however, don't get caught up on other people's dieting stories and nightmares, focus on your own. Ask yourself some honest questions about your current diet and be real with your answers and write them down! It can be a great exercise to review these later on.

Start with these suggested questions:

- How many calories a day do I normally consume?

- How much is protein?

- How much is fat?

- How much are carbohydrates?

- Of these carbs, how many are complex and how many are simple?

- When do I typically eat less healthy items?

- When do I normally eat healthier?

- How much do I weigh and what is my ideal weight?

Just looking at and analyzing your diet from a caloric and nutritional viewpoint can have a dramatic impact on your health and longevity. You will likely discover yourself avoiding or limiting fat promoting foods for a long time after you stop carb cycling, simply because you're now aware of how they impact your body.

If possible, it is suggested you visit your doctor and have some blood tests done to determine what your body fat levels are and ask your doctor what an ideal body fat percentage would be for someone like you. Doctors like to speak in general terms when discussing things like ideal body weight, but ask your doctor what your ideal weight target would be. This is also a good opportunity to be tested for vitamin and mineral deficiencies, as you can address these at the same time you're figuring out the other aspects. Whether you address any deficiencies by increasing a number of nutritional foods in your diet or via supplements, it is valuable information to know.

All of this information will come in very handy when you begin to set a carb cycling regimen for yourself. Once you know where you will be starting from, you can take this information and use it to begin measuring results.

Once you have documented where you will be starting from, it is then time to focus on the changes you plan on making to your diet. This can be a fun exercise because it really forces you to focus on the healthy aspects of your diet. You will absolutely begin to look at food in an entirely different light. Instead of seeing a potato, you'll see 200 calories of carbs and a two-mile walk to burn it off.

A good number to start with when mapping out your carb cycling plan is the ten percent rule. Remember, you can't set a realistic number of calories and carbohydrates as a goal until you've determined what your caloric baseline is. This baseline is the number of calories that you need to simply maintain your weight, or in other words, the amount of calories you burn away on any given day.

These following numbers are only for easy mathematical calculations and are not intended as advised targets.

If a 2000 calorie diet is your baseline number, then your carb cycling plan should start at ten percent less, or 1800 calories per day. Taking those 1800 calories, you then want to divide that into the three categories of fat, protein, and carbs.

Briefly revisiting the 4-9-4 rule, carbs and proteins yield approximately four calories per gram, while fat yields approximately nine calories per gram so it will look something like this:

Target for total daily calories is 1800

- Fat-180 calories (10% of total) or 20 grams

- Protein-630 calories (35% of total) or 158 grams

- Carbs-990 calories (55% of total) or 248 grams

There are 454 grams in one pound, so the diet above would total 426 grams of food daily or just under one pound.

You would then divide those 1800 calories into breakfast, lunch, and dinner. You could also drop to two meals a day and split things up or even spread it out over meals and snacks throughout the day. This is all based on personal preference, and only you can decide what works and what doesn't.

If you are very active in the morning, it makes sense to beef up that portion of your day with a higher percentage of calories, particularly the carbs, since that's where most of your energy comes from. Thinking about it in these terms will help you decide where you can best allocate your calories throughout the day.

It is never too early to start this process, and the sooner you get this done, the closer you are to being on tour way to a trimmer, healthier self.

Chapter 10
Creating Your Own Customized Carb Cycles

A magical formula that everyone can follow and watch the fat melt away does not exist. Not in a carb cycling diet, not in any diet. What works for someone who has a similar weight, height, and lifestyle as you might produce completely different results.

You can always use the philosophy of a certain diet to work towards your own, but never expect someone else's successful diet recipe to work for everybody. There are simply too many nuances. It's one of the things that makes life interesting, that we are all unique in our own way.

It was stated previously that carb cycling is a complex diet which requires planning, setting goals, making commitments and sticking to them, while also making slight adjustments along the way. The variables are plenty, the moving parts are countless, and every single person will have a different result after completing a carb cycling regimen.

What we can do, however, is show you some examples of what successful carb cycling diets look like, how they are laid out, break them down into sections and guide you along to set up your own customized plan.

The key words here are 'customized plan,' because dieting and exercise are as unique as people. You cannot describe people without pointing to their unique quirks and qualities, and so this goes with diets. There is no one size that fits all.

Over a seven-day week, the most common carb cycle calendars start with a low carb day. It may look something like this:

- Mon - Low Carb

- Tue - Med Carb

- Wed - Low Carb

- Thu - Med Carb

- Fri - Low Carb

- Sat - Med Carb

- Sun - Hi Carb

This would normally be in conjunction with a regular workout schedule where an individual would want to exercise on the medium and high carb days while resting on the low carb days. This is also assuming you are going to include an exercise regimen in your diet.

It is highly recommended that you write out your daily schedule first, including workout days and then wrap your carb cycling around that. This way, you aren't killing yourself trying to change your entire life around a diet but rather changing your diet to fit your life. You will find this greatly increases your likelihood of success.

One of the wonderful things about carb cycling is that you can change the order of low and medium carb days any way you like, without disrupting important routines. You may discover that starting your week off with a high carb day works best for you and provides the energy you need to get through the week. Or perhaps inserting your high carb day into the middle of the week to help get you over the hump.

Keep in mind that the above example is just that, an example. Some people have success with two high carb days while alternating the remaining five. Basically, whatever floats your boat. There is no need to stick to a rotation that is clearly not working for you, so plan on trying different rotations until you find the one that will get you to your target.

This also applies to an exercise schedule, depending on how committed you are. Some body builders tough out their exercise schedules where the hardest workouts are completed on the low carb days in order to maximize fat loss while increasing muscle tone. Remember, the sugar in your blood is the first to get used, not the energy stored as body fat.

A standard rule of thumb, when exercising, is that during the first twenty minutes of heavy activity, your body is pulling its energy directly from your bloodstream. After that, your body begins to burn stored fat, so make sure you are scheduling your gym time accordingly. There's little point in working out for only twenty minutes at a time because you want to get that body fat burning off. This applies to any type of exercise, be it swimming, running, lifting weights, whatever.

Hopefully, now you have a good idea of what a carb cycling calendar looks like, and you're comfortable with setting up your own customized diet.

Chapter 11
Meet Average Bob (A Parable, Of All Sorts)

Let's introduce you, Bob. He is a fictional character, but you might know someone just like him.

Bob is an average person in the most average of ways. He's a little short of six feet tall, weighs a very average of 185 lbs. and carries around your average beer belly, disguised as a spare tire. Over the past couple of years, Bob has picked up around twenty pounds, and it all came after his promotion to a desk job at work. Prior to that, he had always maintained a trim figure and hovered close to 165 lbs. so he never paid any attention to his weight.

Now, all of that is changing.

He is approaching middle age, and he recently went through a divorce, so all of a sudden, Bob has decided he needs to shed some weight, lose some body fat and tone up his muscles a bit. Everybody knows a Bob in their life.

Should Bob dive head first, into a carb cycling diet? The short answer is no. The best thing Bob can do is slowly work his way towards it. His first step should be focused on looking at his lifestyle objectively and do a self-review. Basically, he should identify his starting line and set goals from there.

The first thing Bob did was to begin weighing himself daily and started writing down what he eats. He then measured his meals and converted that information into calories. It turns out that he consumes an average of 3000 calories a day.

Since he knew he'd been picking up an extra pound or so every month, one of the early things he changed was how many calories he ingested on a daily basis, dropping them down to 2700 calories. A simple ten percent reduction in food for a little while.

It wasn't enough of a change to leave him hungry, which was a surprise, but it did stop him from continuing to gain weight. So Bob now knew that his caloric baseline was right around 2700 calories. Step one was accomplished.

Bob had set a goal for himself to lose twenty pounds but he also wanted to lose it all from his belly area and not anywhere else. He also wanted to tone his muscles up a little, so he knew there would be an exercise commitment involved.

Next, Bob took a look at what exactly he was eating and where his calories were coming from. It turned out that his usual diet consisted of 75% carbohydrates and just 25% of protein and fat. So he made some changes and increased his total fats and proteins to 45% and reduced his carbs to 65%.

He also stopped drinking soda and started to put less sugar in his coffee, along with reducing his daily donut to only once or twice per week. Basically, he reduced or eliminated junk food and processed foods from his diet.

Also, since he was focused on shrinking his waist line, Bob began an exercise routine where he focused mainly on the stomach area, doing a lot of sit ups. This turned out to be quite significant because by using the stomach area muscles, those were the first to tighten up and also the body fat that had accumulated into a spare tire was the first body fat to begin burning away.

Even though he continued to consume 2700 calories per day, he began to drop weight and noticed his gut was tightening up a little. This happened just by reducing his simple carbohydrate consumption and increasing his fat and protein.

In two weeks, he lost five pounds with a minimal effort, and he hadn't even gone to the gym yet! He had only been doing sit ups at home until this point. Bob thought he was golden until the weight loss stopped dead in its tracks. He had hit a full 25% of his weight loss target in two weeks but made the mistake of assuming it would just continue. It didn't. What he lost was mostly water weight and not actual body fat.

Water weight is always the first thing to go and the easiest weight to lose.

Increased exercise would have helped him a little, but even that would have only delayed the brick wall by a short period of time. This is where Bob decided to dig into a carb cycling diet and really make a commitment to changing his food and exercise lifestyle.

The important thing that Bob had discovered was that consuming 2700 calories per day was still too high for him to reach his goal, but at least he had enough information now to make further adjustments.

Fearful of taking his carb cycling too far and too fast, Bob decided to drop a further 5% off his daily caloric intake, bringing it down to 2575 in total. He also started alternating med to low carb days with medium to high carb days. He did this because he knew himself well enough to realize a high carb cheat day would be too enticing to avoid gorging.

He kept the same ratios of fats, proteins, and carbs overall, but dropped half of them one day, followed by a double ration the next. He also increased his daily sit up routine by five percent as well. It did not take long for him to notice a couple of dramatic changes and soon realized some additional adjustments were in order.

Until now, he had been taking his calories in equal parts across breakfast, lunch, and dinner, while doing his sit ups first thing in the morning. The problem was that he was simply starving well before dinner time and consumed by thoughts of food and occasional hunger pangs. He couldn't focus on anything else, and this was a problem.

To try and combat this, he moved his sit up routine to the evenings, shortly before dinner, and also took some of his morning and lunch calories and also moved them to the evening. Another important adjustment he made was moving a larger chunk of his daily carb ration to dinner as well, leaving mostly protein and fat to lunch and breakfast. This produced a pleasant surprise. His hunger pangs went away in the afternoon, and he was no longer distracted by thoughts of food for, what seemed, hours on end.

Let's take a look at why these minor changes helped Bob with his carb cycling.

The first issue Bob had gotten himself into was the gap between dinner and breakfast which resulted in him exercising on a completely empty stomach. When he did eat breakfast, those calories disappeared quickly into his system, trying to recover from his sit up routine. In hindsight, he should have eaten a larger breakfast and reduced his lunch and dinner calories. He also should have consumed more carbohydrates closer to his workout and lowered his carbs later in the day. This would have reduced his overwhelming sense of hunger later in the day. The adjustments Bob made also began to show some surprising results in muscle tone as the six pack abs he hadn't seen since high school, were showing signs of returning.

What happened here is that Bob had discovered, by pure accident and luck, 'backloading,' a fairly new take on carb cycling, and one that is proving to be a highly effective muscle toning strategy. This leads us to the next chapter on back loading carbohydrates.

Chapter 12
'Backloading' Your Carbohydrates

Up until this point, everything you have read in this book has revolved around limiting the amount of calories you consume – avoiding this, eating less of that, carbs are bad, count, count, count and on and on.

That is all about to change as we delve into the realm of dietary bliss, also known as back loading. The concept of back loading carbohydrates is a relatively new approach to dieting for body fat loss, and the discovery of this system can be attributed to a gentleman named John Kiefer.

Kiefer is quite well known throughout the dieting, body building and exercise worlds, so it might surprise you to discover that his background is in physics. The scientific universe of physics is not one that frequently crosses paths with the world of barbells and cardiovascular workouts. However, this is exactly what has happened, and this galactic sized collision of science and exercise has resulted in one of the most effective, yet counter intuitive dietary approaches, in the history of dietary approaches. This is known as 'Carb Back Loading,' or simply CBL.

Utilizing his knowledge of science, nutrition, and exercise, combined with the understanding that people just like to eat, Mr. Kiefer has created a full on revolution in the way people think about shedding body fat without suffering through a miserable diet. To a certain degree, at least. However, the results speak for themselves.

Although CBL can be considered a unique dietary philosophy, there is no question that its roots are firmly planted in the ground of carb cycling. In fact, it is carb cycling, but with a twist.

In previous chapters, we have covered the significance of how cycling your carbohydrate consumption changes the way your body burns stored energy, and we have referenced examples what this cycling might look like. There is no question that cycling carbs will reduce your body fat without compromising muscle strength. However Mr. Kiefer has discovered that taking things a step further will not only continue to produce these same results, but it will also allow you to continue eating what you enjoy while doing so. The bottom line is, with a back loading approach, you don't have to avoid foods you love. There is a simple reason why so many people are overweight, beyond a general lack of exercise; we love our carbs!

Yes, you are going to need to continue counting your calories, and yes, you will still need to schedule some time in the gym, however, in this case, there can still be a nice large plate of your favorite pasta waiting at the end of the day.

The basic premise of a carbohydrate back loaded program is that instead of spreading your daily carb allowance over breakfast, lunch, and dinner, or even two of the three meals, you focus on packing all of your daily carbs into one large meal. This would include all three components of a carb cycling regimen, meaning you take the same approach on a low or medium carb day as you would the high carb day.

The caveat is that the daily meal with all your carb rations is also your last meal of the day, so in its most basic form, a back loaded diet means that protein and fat are the only foods you consume in the morning and afternoon.

Timing is also important with a back loaded diet as the effectiveness of burning off body fat and driving excess sugars to your muscles instead of your gut requires consuming those carbohydrates at a specific time in your day. It also requires consistency.

In order for this approach to work effectively to burn off body fat, you will still need a detailed daily and weekly plan, you will still need to count your calories and manage your total carb intake, and you will still want to engage in a regular exercise routine. It is not like these requirements will magically disappear. That is not how any diet works.

Having said that, keep in mind that if you are an amateur dieter who just wants to lose a few pounds, or reduce your body fat a little, a carb cycling diet can and will work for you. This also includes a back loaded approach, just don't expect six pack abs and runway models dropping at your feet. Keep your expectations real.

So, what exactly would a backloaded, carb cycled diet look like on any given day?

For now, let's assume Bob is going to the gym every afternoon to spend a couple of hours working on cardio. We will also assume that Bob has decided he is comfortable with his current weight status of 165 lbs.

Through trial and error, he discovered that 2800 calories per day, on average, combined with regular exercise is the perfect number to maintain his body weight. Without regular exercise, he also knows he needs to drop his calorie intake to 2400 calories per day, but that leaves him hungry sometimes, so he'd rather commit to the gym on a regular basis and enjoy his food.

Even though he is comfortable with his current weight, he is still carrying that spare tire around and would rather burn that body fat down, or more preferably, convert it to muscle. So here we are, spending an hour or two at the gym every day. Bob hasn't felt this energetic and fit since his college football days. Therefore this has become a pretty compelling routine that he sees no reason to quit.

Since Bob is fortunate enough to work for himself, he has the luxury of setting his work schedule around his personal life. A day in the life of Bob looks something like this:

- 6 AM Wake up

- 7 AM Coffee, no sugar

- 8 AM 20 minutes run to get going for the day

- 9 AM Breakfast of two eggs and two ounces of cheese

- 11 AM Protein shake and daily vitamin regimen

- 1 PM Lunch of 6oz ground beef or steak, 8 ounces of milk, 2 ounces of cheese

- 3 PM Workout at the gym for two hours

- 5 PM Protein shake,

- 6 PM Dinner time!

At dinner, Bob eats pretty much whatever he wants, focusing on high carbs, mostly the complex carbs. However he does enjoy an occasional dessert and the simple carbs that come with the package. His dinner usually contains around six ounces of lean protein, a generous portion of starch, (pasta, potatoes, dinner rolls, etc.) and as many green vegetables as he can eat. He has gotten so good at this through practice, he barely counts his calories anymore, since he's been doing this for a while. In other words, after just a few weeks of measuring his calories and managing fat, protein and carb intakes, he nails his diet on a regular basis. Of course, his diet app has helped with this to a large degree.

The breakdown you see above is one of Bob's medium to high carb days. As a general rule, he drops his carbs by 30 percent on any day he can't make it to the gym and maintains his regular carb cycling routine. This has become an exception for him though since the back loading program and exercise commitment have negated his low carb days.

The following is an outline, in layman's terms, of how a carbohydrate, back loaded diet works internally to burn your body fat and prevent the carb calories from becoming body fat in the first place.

By now, you should be aware that fat and protein do not provide your body with energy like carbs do. Remember, simple carbs put sugar in your blood for instant energy and if not used immediately, head directly to your body fat. Complex carbs do the same thing, only slower, as they take longer to break down and digest. By avoiding the consumption of these, soon to be sugars and body fat, during the daytime hours, your body has no choice but to pull its energy from your body fat instead of your bloodstream.

Of course, this does put some stresses on your body as it searches for available body fat to convert to the energy you may need in any given task, and this includes simple digestion. Most of this body fat is pulled from the places near where the muscles you are using for said task reside. For example, if you are doing sit ups, the body fat is being drawn from your middle section. Squats will pull from your legs and so on.

To sidebar here for a moment, this is one of the most obvious benefits of carb cycling and back loading your diet. You can literally focus on one single part of your body that you want to improve, and once you get there, you're able to move on to other areas.

By depriving your bloodstream of easily available sugars, the excess body fat is the first to go, followed by any fat available in the muscles you are using. This is part of the magic of the back loaded strategy because when you do sit down for dinner, the carbohydrates you are enjoying, along with the sugars and starches they contain, head right for the muscles and places your body needs them. In essence, they are being pulled from your digestive system and bloodstream and immediately put to work, as opposed to gravitating their way into your waist line or what have you.

This is the essence of back loaded carbohydrates; when you do consume carbs after exercising, but avoid them before exercising, those carbohydrate sugars go to where you want them to, rather than where they are used to going. The same is true for carb cycling in general.

There are loads upon loads of biological and chemical reactions involved in this process, including complex details involving fructose versus glucose and insulin and many other intricate interactions which are scientific in nature. These types of metabolic reactions and digestive endeavors are highly technical and complicated to explain, let alone understand. A beginner's guide to carb cycling for body fat loss is not the proper vehicle for this type of information, and we have little desire to overwhelm the reader with information that may complicate the understanding of this type of diet. Specifically, our goal is to keep things as simple as possible so that readers can garner enough information to make informed decisions as to whether this type of diet is worth exploring further. There is a plethora of information available both online and in print which can take the reader as far into the dieting rabbit hole as one may choose to delve.

Chapter 13
Does Carb Cycling Work Without Exercise?

Will carb cycling be effective as a diet for weight for fat loss, even without exercise?

The short answer is yes. However, the results will not be achieved as quickly as they would in tandem with an exercise program. Earlier in this book, we discussed to origins of carb cycling being traced back to the professional body building industry of the 1980's. Obviously, it was originally designed as part of an overall strategy to maximize the physical presentation of developed muscles during competition.

Also, due to the nature of carb cycling being designed to tax your metabolism, this is a dietary approach which was never meant to become a permanent lifestyle change. Therefore, since a maximum of nine weeks is the window for carb cycling, taking on this diet without exercising will never achieve the same level of results as it would with exercise.

When resting and even while sleeping, your body is burning calories with every heartbeat and every breath. The fundamental principles still apply, where carb cycling reduces the available sugars for energy in your blood stream, forcing your body to burn stored fat instead.

However, if your goal is to reduce some body fat by just changing your eating habits for a limited period of time, then yes, carb cycling is certainly worth a try. Just don't expect to magically beef up your chest muscles by altering what and when you eat.

One of the more beneficial side effects of undertaking a carb cycling challenge is once you start paying close attention to what you eat, it tends to become a habit you carry on with, even after you've finished the diet. Naturally, this can lead to a healthier lifestyle for the long term.

Conclusion

Losing excess body fat and improving overall health is a goal everyone aspires to. It is rarely easy and never successful without effort. Carb cycling has helped millions of people over the years, to achieve their weight loss goals while also improving muscle tone and strength.

Although this dieting movement was founded by people involved in professional body building, it is the type of diet that can help anyone who desires to change their diet for the better. This is not a diet exclusive to any group of people.

We understand that a carb cycling diet may not be for everyone. However, we certainly strived to present enough information for anybody to be able to make an informed decision as to whether carb cycling is something worth trying or exploring further. The brutal truth is that there is an overwhelming amount of information available and much of it is conflicting. Even the medical community is at odds as to whether carb cycling and other carb reduced diets are healthy or not.

Perhaps you have heard the expression; "There is more than one way to get to New York.", inferring diet plans which prove effective for some people, simply have little positive results for others. When considering whether carb cycling is a good diet choice or not, the very first thing you need to understand is that all diets are more of an art than a science. Every individual who attempts any diet regimen is endeavoring on a brand new experiment, in and of itself. This fact must not be ignored.

Of course, science is applied to the theory of dieting, particularly more so over the past two decades, however, real science only works in a world of absolutes. Science, by definition, is a process which can be proven, time and time again, by following an exact same protocol. If a protocol is followed exactly, the results produced will be exactly the same every single time. This is where scientific theory becomes scientific fact.

When the human body becomes part of the scientific protocol, results in a dietary sense can never be exactly the same as no two subjects are the same, to begin with. This is why you never see a government sanctioned diet that guarantees specific results if specific procedures are followed. This is also why all diets for fat loss are spoken of in general terms, and you never see a claim of guaranteed results.

If you ever encounter a claim of certain results by any diet, it will only be a matter of time before a lawsuit for false advertising is filed. Understand though, it's not just the diet, it's you, and it is also the food you eat. Two people can undertake the exact same diet plan together, in tandem, and experience different results, different side effects, even down to one body absorbing more nutrients than another, while eating the exact same thing.

Carb cycling is no exception, and this can be both a good thing and potentially, a bad thing. The message we are trying to drive home is one of trial and error, tweaks and adjustments and listening to the messages your body sends you. Regardless of how well a diet works for one person, never expect those same results yourself. Be flexible, remain that way and pay close attention to the messages your body sends you along the way.

This is especially true during a carb cycling regimen because your metabolism goes through changes that it hasn't likely experienced before. Therefore unintended consequences can always be right around the corner.

We'd like to thank you for making it through to the end of this book. We understand it is a lot of reading and a broad array of information and insight was covered as thoroughly as possible. While trying to avoid overloading you with more information than you need, we tried diligently to provide you with as much relevant and compelling information as possible.

We certainly hope you enjoyed your reading experience and found this information useful and inspiring. More importantly, we hope you found the information in this book usable in your quest for a healthier lifestyle.

Another goal was to enable people who are considering a carb cycling diet to develop a clear sense of what is involved and what can be achieved. If you agree, feel free to let your friends know this book is available. If you found this book useful, informative and a fun read, a positive review on Amazon is always appreciated!